HOMEMADE FACE MASK

Step By Step Guide To Make Your Own Different Types Of Reusable Medical Face Mask To Protect Yourself From Viruses.

Josephine Samlace

© Copyright 2020 by Josephine Samlace

All rights reserved.

This document is geared towards providing exact and reliable information with regards to the topic and issue covered. The publication is sold with the idea that the publisher is not required to render accounting, officially permitted, or otherwise, qualified services. If advice is necessary, legal or professional, a practiced individual in the profession should be ordered.

From a Declaration of Principles which was accepted and approved equally by a Committee of the American Bar Association and a Committee of Publishers and Associations.

In no way is it legal to reproduce, duplicate, or transmit any part of this document in either electronic means or in printed format. Recording of this publication is strictly prohibited and any storage of this document is not allowed unless with written permission from the publisher. All rights reserved.

The information provided herein is stated to be truthful and consistent, in that any liability, in terms of inattention or otherwise, by any usage or abuse of any policies, processes, or directions contained within is the solitary and utter responsibility of the recipient reader. Under no circumstances will any legal responsibility or blame be held against the publisher for any reparation, damages, or monetary loss due to the information herein, either directly or indirectly.

Respective authors own all copyrights not held by the publisher.

The information herein is offered for informational purposes solely, and is universal as so. The presentation of the information is without contract or any type of guarantee assurance.

The trademarks that are used are without any consent, and the publication of the trademark is without permission or backing by the trademark owner. All trademarks and brands within this book are for clarifying purposes only and are the owned by the owners themselves, not affiliated with this document.

DISCLAIMER

This book details the author's personal experiences with and opinions about Homemade Masks.

The author is not your healthcare provider.

The author and publisher are providing this book and its contents on an "as is" basis and make no representations or warranties of any kind with respect to this book or its contents.

The author and publisher disclaim all such representations and warranties, including for example warranties of merchantability and healthcare for a particular purpose.

In addition, the author and publisher do not represent or warrant that the information accessible via this book is accurate, complete or current.

The statements made about products and services have not been evaluated by the U.S. Food and Drug Administration.

They are not intended to diagnose, treat, cure, or prevent any condition or disease. Please consult with your own physician or healthcare specialist regarding the suggestions and recommendations made in this book.

Except as specifically stated in this book, neither the author or publisher, nor any authors, contributors, or other representatives will be liable for damages arising out of or in connection with the use of this book.

This is a comprehensive limitation of liability that applies to all damages of any kind, including (without limitation) compensatory; direct, indirect or consequential damages; loss of data, income or profit; loss of or damage to property and claims of third parties.

You understand that this book is not intended as a substitute for consultation with a licensed healthcare practitioner, such as your physician. Before you begin any healthcare program, or change your lifestyle in any way, you will consult your physician or another licensed healthcare practitioner to ensure that you are in good health and that the examples contained in this book will not harm you.

This book provides content related to physical and/or mental health issues.

As such, use of this book implies your acceptance of this disclaimer.

TABLE OF CONTENTS

Introduction III
Chapter 1: Introduction 1
   What Exactly A Face Mask Is? 2
   History Of Facemasks 3
   Are Facemasks Effective? 4
Chapter 2: Types Of Facemasks 7
   Surgical Masks 7
   N95 Mask 8
   Cloth Mask 10
   Use Of Facemasks Prior Covid-19 11
   Use Of Facemasks After Covid-19 11
Chapter 3: Why Homemade Face Masks? 13
   How Effective Are Diy Face Masks? 15
   Can Just Using Face Mask Protect Me From Covid-19? 16
   Who And Hand Sanitization 17
   Cdc And Social Distancing 18
   China And Precautionary Measures 19
   Other Countries 20
   Face Mask Or Face Covering? 21
Chapter 4: Factors To Look For 22
   1.   Breathable 22
   2.   Filtration Power 23
   3.   Face Shapes 24
   4.   Ear Protection 25
   Materials: Which One To Go For 25
   1.   Pillowcases 25
   2.   Flannel Pajamas 26
   3.   Kitchen Towels 26

- 4. Bedsheets 26
- 5. Quilters Cotton 27
- Materials: Which One To Avoid 27
  - 1. Vacuum Cleaner Bags 27
  - 2. Old T-Shirts 28
  - 3. Fiberglass Fabrics 28
  - 4. Regular Cotton 29
- Emergency Materials 29
  - 1. Tissues 29
  - 2. Scarfs 30
  - 3. Bandanas 30
- Chart On Materials 31
- Good Materials 31
- Bad Materials 31
- Emergency Materials 31

Chapter 5: Step By Step Tutorial To Stitch Mask 32
- Material Required 32
- Tools Required 32
- Instructions: 33
- Step By Step Tutorials To Make A No-Sew Mask 37
  - 1. T-Shirt / Flannel Pajama Mask 37
- Materials Required 38
- Tools Required 38
- Instructions 38
- 2 Bandana Face Mask 41
- Materials Required 41
- Tools Required 42
- Instructions 42
- Bandana Face Mask Using A Coffee Filter 44
- Important Notes 45

Chapter 6: What Is The Proper Way To Wear A Mask? 47
What Is The Proper Way To Un-Wear A Mask? 48
Common Mistakes About Masks 49
1. Thinking Not Wearing A Mask Is Okay! 49
2. Occasionally Wearing A Mask 49
3. Not Washing Hands Before Or After Using A Mask 49
4. Wearing Loose Masks 49
5. Wearing Too Tight Masks 50
6. Touching The Mask After Wearing It 50
7. Un-Wearing The Face Mask From The Front Part 51
8. Hanging The Mask Around The Neck 51
9. Hanging The Mask From One Ear 51
10. Reusing A Mask Without Washing It Properly 51

Frequently Asked Questions Regarding Masks 52
1. Should A Face Mask Cover The Chin? 52
2. How To Touch Mask After Wearing It? 52
3. How Frequently Should The Mask Be Replaced? 52
4. What To Do If The Ears Get Rashes Or Redness? 52
5. What Are The Places You Should Wear A Mask? 53
6. What About The Small Gaps In Masks? 53
7. Which One Is Better: Stitched Or Non-Stitched Masks? 53
8. Should You Wear A Mask At Home? 54
9. What If You Have To Un-Wear A Mask? 54
10. What Are The Quick Dos And Don'ts Of Wearing Masks? ... 54

Bottom Line 55

References 56

CHAPTER 1
INTRODUCTION

Learning how to make a face mask was not at all important a year ago. It was precisely the job of those related to health care only. No one had thought of it until we all met with something that shattered our lives and ruined our freedom to live. The pandemic started from the heart of China, Wuhan has now reached almost every corner of the globe, with the number of deaths rising each day.

The safety precautions are still there, trying to save the mother earth from the disaster, but the situation is getting worse. This is a time of crisis, and staying silent is not a condition. All across the planet, the cities are vacant, and hospitals are full of patients. More than two hundred and fifty-two thousand deaths, not within a year, seem impossible. But it is happening, and people are dying, with every second. As an outcome, the precautionary measures are must to follow, for the safety of humanity, and the mother earth.

Since there is no vaccine or antidote, the fears are multiplying. And the only way to be safe in such a time of danger is to follow precautions. A facemask may seem a tiny thing, but it can and has prevented the spread of deadly viruses. This simple piece of fabric daily used by health care workers has now become so significant that without it, it is impossible to breathe safely. All parts of the words are equally suffering, and in a situation like this where going out is nearly out of reach, the best is to stay home and prepare hand-crafted facemasks.

What exactly a face mask is?

A face mask can mean many things at one time, cosmetic treatment, respirator, and even a hood. But here we are, precisely talking about a covering that is worn over the mouth and nose. In the world of etymology, the word "mask" was derived from Italian "Maschera" and from medieval Latin "masca," which primarily meant "specter." The term made its appearance in English from Middle French "masque" and was intended to mean anything that could "hide or guard the face."

A facemask is made with different materials, and in the modern world, it is typically used to protect the face from dust and other harmful microorganisms. It is a re-useable covering first designed to avoid the dissemination of pathogens and infections during operations and surgeries. The one who wears a mask is protected not only from debris but also from harmful droplets and bacteria hanging in the air.

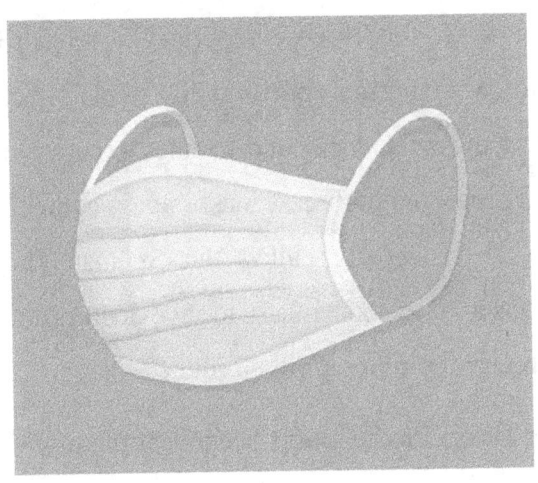

One thing to note is that the mask does not cause the inhalation of microorganisms as the material used for the preparation is too wide to avoid any pores that could allow the passing of viruses. Since the mouth and nose are the most open sources of getting any pathogen inside the body, the mask effectively terminates the crossing of any particle into the wearer's mouth and nose.

History of facemasks

Facemasks were not conventional in the past. They were originated in 1897 by a French surgeon Paul Berger, who was a practitioner in Paris. He marked the history with the use of first cloth masks during the pneumonic epidemic at the beginning of the 20th century. While the world was suffering from an infectious disease, Wu Lien-Teh, a Malaysian doctor, designed a mask to protect the health care professionals from pathogens and microorganisms during the outbreak of Manchurian pneumonic plague.

Those who served the Chinese Imperial Court from 1910 to 1911 and till the Manchurian pneumonic plague settled started acknowledging masks that inspired its later generation. Just after a few years of pneumonia outbreak, masks again came into due to the pandemic in 1918, mostly called the Spanish flu. Afterward, cheesecloth was used to make masks to save doctors and nurses from the toxic pathogens of tuberculosis in the 1940s.

During the 1960s, clothe masks became popular with their ability to filter out any dangerous particles. Following upon, they were replaced by surgical masks that were explicitly designed for those involved in medicine. These masks used nonwoven fabric, and their fine filtration of microorganisms made them handy and preferable. Because surgical masks were costly, cloth masks were still used in developing states, precisely during the SARS outbreak in Asia from 2002-4 as well as during the Ebola pandemic in West Africa since the 2013-16.

Are facemasks effective?

In 1918, there was the first research on the usage of masks for healthcare personnel. However, not much observational research analysis or guidelines on face masks had been performed since then. Some work had been undertaken in the early 20th century before that was before the emergence of surgical masks. CR MacIntyre, in his study in 2010, explained that facemasks could lead to personal hygiene by preventing viruses and pathogens from entering the human body.

The effectiveness of any face masks depends on the material. Different materials have different filtration abilities, and factors such as design, a number of layers, or the fitness over the face also play their role, and thus the effectiveness of one face mask varies from the other. Whatever the material or design is, however, the primary purpose is to stop the dissemination of viruses.

In 2013, an experiment by Anna Davies was performed to check the strength of facemasks. The materials used were nonwoven fabric, vacuum cleaner bag, a cotton t-shirt, and a tea towel bag. The results validated the reliable filtration of surgical masks as the nonwoven fabric filtered 90% of the virus particles in the air. While, the vacuum cleaner bag refined only 89%, the cotton t-shirt only 51%, and the tea-towel only 72% of contaminants. Thus, masks are beneficial when it comes to the safety and prevention of pathogens.

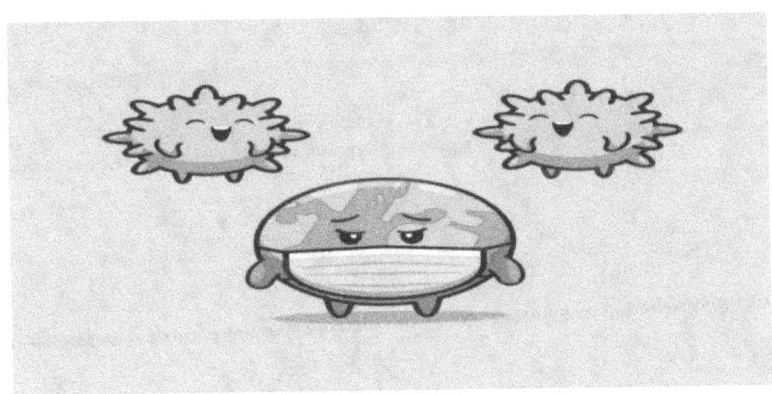

Apart from that, in the modern world, facemasks are highly encouraged to help prevent the dissemination of COVID-19. The Centers of Disease Control and Prevention, CDC, has recommended the use of face masks to all healthcare professionals while dealing with sick patients, especially those infected with flu. The CDC has also put stress on providing masks to those who display symptoms.

CHAPTER 2
TYPES OF FACEMASKS

We've been learning a lot about face masks over the last few months. From an international lack of masks to the new CDC guidelines urging more residents to wear fabric masks in public spaces, and to take steps to give face masks to vulnerable healthcare organizations, there is no question face masks have made their place in the top of our priorities. If talk about their types, well, there are three, and the difference comes in the material and the way each type is prepared.

Surgical masks

Surgical masks are made with nonwoven fabric. This type of masks is disposable, meaning it cannot be used again and should be thrown once they become wet with saliva, sweat, or other body fluids. It has a loose-fitting and serves as a hindrance in the way of the wearer's mouth and the nose. When a person wears a surgical mask, the harmful contaminants, impurities, or other pollutants remain outside the boundary created by the mask, and thus, they cannot enter the body. Any type of droplet, splash, pathogen, bacteria, or virus in the air sticks to its surface and stays away from the mouth and nose.

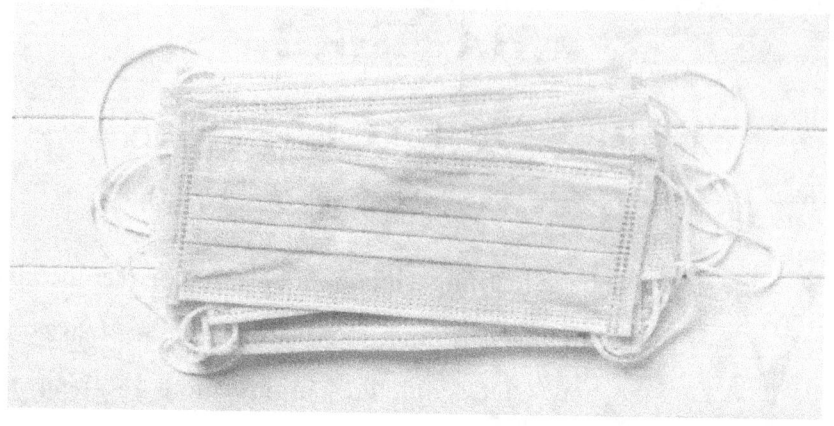

It is worth noting that surgical masks are also useful not only in preventing pollutants and impurities in the air from reaching the wearer's mouth and nose, but also, they help in reducing the possibility of wearer's saliva and other respiratory emissions from getting exposed to a harmful environment. In simple terms, they work both ways and are quite useful.

However, what should not be ignored is the loose fit between the face and mask. If surgical masks are not worn out appropriately, they fail to protect the body from pathogens and other impurities. Also, surgical masks are designed in such a way that they cannot filter minimal impurities in the air that can lead to transmission of illness through sneezes or coughs. This is precisely why the CDC has not recommended people wear surgical masks.

N95 mask

This is another popular form of masks. In N95, the 'N' refers to "not resistant to oil," because the mask defends only against oils, and no fluids. While, "95" indicates that by using this mask, almost

95% of the airborne contaminants and impurities will be washed out. In simple terms, an N95 mask is a particle size-filtering face-shield respirator that removes at least 95% of pathogenic organisms, although not oil-impurities.

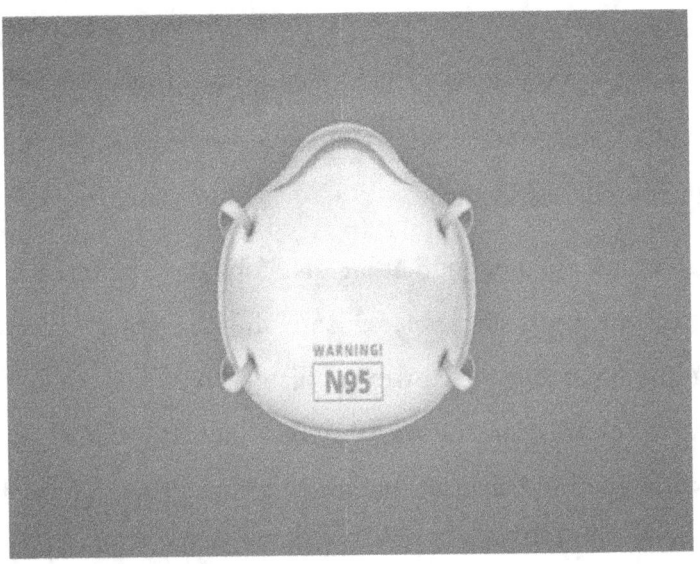

N95 mask is good for filtration of pollutants, the N95 mask is constructed of nonwoven fabric, typically polypropylene plastic. In comparison with surgical masks, it prefers equal protection to the body as it effectively stops a large number of contaminants in the air. Since these masks provide too much security, they are used in hospitals by physicians, nurses, and those who look after infected patients.

As far as the CDC is concerned, it has not prescribed surgical masks to be used by the public, mainly because these should be worn by those prone to viruses directly. Also, due to the shortage in their availability and the fact that it is nearly impossible to supply N95 masks to all the people across the globe, CDC has recommended everyone to preserve these for health care professionals only.

Cloth mask

The last one is the cloth face mask. It is the most common type of facemask in routine use. The material used to prepare a cloth mask is typically cotton, and like all other types of masks, it is worn over the mouth and the nose.

It is commonly thought that the main objective behind the fabric masks is to keep the wearer safe from getting infected or transmitting pathogens. However, history has proved that cloth masks were also in use in the old days to defect medical professionals from bacterial illnesses, such as those in Manchurian pneumonic in 1910 and 1918 Spanish flu. They were replaced by surgical masks in the 1960s; however, they were still used in the least developed countries.

With the outbreak of Covid-19, cloth face masks are back in demand. In places where it is challenging to maintain social isolation, that is six feet apart, such as in supermarkets or clinics, people are highly advised by the CDC to use fabric face masks. Some people are using a scarf or any other fabric to just wrap it around their mouth and nose. However, there are also ways to make face masks at home. The only thing that matters is the thick layer, just like surgical or N95 masks, to ensure the prevention of pathogens.

Use of facemasks prior COVID-19

Since face masks have been acknowledged all across the globe, prior to COVID-19, they were in use only by medical staff or infected patients. Also, surgical facemasks were highly popular, and cloth face masks were used only in third world countries. Though cloth face masks cannot compete with the flexibility and protection of surgical and N95 masks, they can be reused and recycled. Thus, they were used as a "gate protection" on those who were infected with any disease to prevent spread illness by any means. Also, as a reasonable alternative to surgical or N95 masks, they were highly used by doctors and nurses when the other types of masks were out of reach.

Use of facemasks after COVID-19

The history has seen a sudden increase in the need for cloth face masks due to the shortages of surgical and N95 masks. Everyone is encouraged to use fabric face masks as much as possible to remain un-infected by COVID-19. Since the replication of COVID-19 happens really fast, and the cases have increased at an alarming rate, the stocks of surgical masks and other respirators have been drained. Seeing that it is nearly impossible to provide everyone in the world with a surgical or N95 mask, the CDC has recommended using cloth face mask instead of any other.

It is noteworthy that just because cloth face masks are reusable, doesn't mean they are less effective than surgical or N95 masks. The only thing that makes them vulnerable is that they need to be washed. In both residential and environmental conditions, they can help prevent the infection and defend against respiratory diseases and air pollutants in the same way surgical and N9 masks. There are different styles of cloth face masks available on the market, but during the health crisis, it is preferable to make hand-crafted facemasks at home.

CHAPTER 3
WHY HOMEMADE FACE MASKS?

Even if the marketplace is full of stylish and colorful face masks, the question is still there that why you should prepare your own face mask. There are several justifications for that. First, it is the time of extreme health crisis, and going out is strictly prohibited by health care professionals. Staying in isolation is mandatory for everyone, not only for their safety but also because it will protect others. What is the benefit of going out of home and shop for a facemask when you can easily make one at home?

Secondly, even if you think you can just go for once, you are highly mistaken. The deadly virus spreads through close communication, and if everyone starts going out even just for one, how would this no-social-distancing prevent the spread of COVID-19. Also, who knows the virus out there may infect you before you reach home? It is not a condition, and everyone must remain in self-isolation at their home to make sure they are safe.

There are also options for purchasing surgical masks or respirators, such as N95. But A, they will require going out, and B, they are in a limited amount, and it is highly recommended to preserve them for medical staff. There are also options for purchasing them online, but fabric clothes are suggested for a reason. They are not reusable like cloth face masks, which means they would be ineffective once they get wet, or contaminated by impurities. Using a homemade cloth face mask is more comfortable to wear, than facing the hectic of using a new surgical or N95 mask every time.

The other point brings us to the shortages of surgical masks or respirators. People are advised to use clothe masks and stay at home so that more-effective masks are used by doctors, nurses, and other health care professionals who spend their days and nights in taking care of infected patients. They are most prone to get sick, and thus, everyone should consider it as their responsibility to use fabric clothes.

Now, you may encounter why a person should wear a mask if all they are doing is to stay at home and remain in isolation. The answer is not tricky. Since the primary source of dissemination of the virus is via air droplets, it can spread really fast if masks are not worn. Whenever a person speaks, there are always droplets coming out of their mouth, and if they are not wearing a mask, they can quickly spread it to others. Also, if the listener is not wearing a mask, the droplets will reach their mouth in no time. They will be protected only if they have a secure layer over their mouth and nose, and that is possible only by using a mask.

How effective are DIY face masks?

There are three basic types of face masks, surgical, N95, and cloth masks. It is generally assumed that due to the material, surgical and N95 are more effective than cloth face masks. But the truth is far away from that. The thing is that it is not the material that prevents a droplet from reaching the mouth and nose, but the layering. Surely material has a part, but how many layers the mask contains has a significant impact on how strong it will be against pathogens and viruses.

The factor of layering plays an important role. A typical cloth mask prevents around 60% to 65% of the particles, so if the layering is doubled, the mask would be able to defend against contaminants in the same way as surgical or N95 masks. Surely there can be a more significant role of material, but given the situations where wrapping a thick piece of fabric may cause difficulties in breathing, it is better to take cloth fabric with two layers.

Also, the material of the face mask is less critical than layering, because thick material may cause you to adjust the mask, whenever your face feels warm. This goes against the precautionary measures that a person should avoid touching their mouth and nose. Besides, there is one more point; everybody is different. Some people find it easy to breathe under blankets, while for some, it is hard to cover their nose due to suffocation. In such a scenario, taking breathes with a shield before nostrils can lead to suffocation. And it may cause a person to remove their mask and taking breaths in air, which again can lead the droplets to enter the body.

All these points are possible to happen, and thus a cloth face mask should be prepared with lots of consideration. Not only the right material, or the right amount of layering should matter, but the fact that everyone has a different face also has a vital part in the preparation of the face mask. An oval face cannot wear a mask that is explicitly designed for a square face, as it will leave space between the surface of the mask and the mouth and nose. Since the main objective of a face mask is to avoid any droplet from entering the body, considerations, and care while preparation is mandatory.

There are simple and easy steps to make effective homemade masks, and if followed appropriately, are more likely to prevent the dissemination of the virus. There are lots of material that can be used to make a cloth face mask such as scarves, towels, bandanas, and handkerchiefs. The only need of the hour is to make it with measurement and adjustments.

Can just using face mask protect me from COVID-19?

The answer is yes, but with conditions. This requires multiple points to justify how a Do It Yourself face mask will protect against deadly coronavirus. None of the health organizations, namely, WHO or CDC, have ensured the single protection of homemade cloth masks. The same goes for Chinese health professionals who have given specific criteria in safety measures. It simply implies that thinking only the use of face mask will protect against viruses is profoundly mistaken.

The face mask is just a part of precautions, and the proper protection will be evaluated with other factors. Everyone should use a mask for safety, but with appropriate, timely hand sanitization, and six feet apart social distancing. The rationale of such a statement will require a handful of recommendations by significant health organizations, including what should be appropriately followed.

WHO and hand sanitization

World Health Organization has highlighted the use of face masks in personal protective measures. It has advised people to use their elbow or any tissue to protect their faces. Also, when they feel cough or sneeze, they should use a tissue and dispose of it quickly after use. Touching the tissue or cloth covering is strictly not recommended, especially the front part which is most exposed to pathogenic organisms.

While WHO has put forward the frequent use of face masks, it has also stated the proper use of hand sanitization for at least 20-30 seconds. Wearing a mask can limit the possibility of getting infected, touching the surface area, and not washing hands can immediately work in the opposite way. Whenever people talk, cough, or sneeze, the droplets travel from their mouth to air. The mask on the other side can stop them, but the hands can only get rid of those droplets by proper sanitization.

WHO has also stated the proper use of masks, to ensure the maximum personal protection, and the effectivity of masks is increased in combination with appropriate hand-washing with a hand sanitizer, soap, or alcohol-based hand wash. People are urged to use hand sanitization after they cough, sneeze, stay in contact with an infected person, and every-time they replace or wash their face masks. Also, though WHO earlier stated that healthy individuals might not need to wear masks, later they have given particular importance to the regular use of face-covering as it can limit the touching of mouth and nose while hand sanitization is required in all cases, whether a person is sick or not.

CDC and social distancing

CDC has frequently recommended people to use face coverings to ensure safety. What CDC has put stress on is that many people are infected before they know they are, which simply entails that a person has no idea who affected and who is not. This increases the danger, and in such a situation where people only wear masks from already-infected patients, it can help spread the virus.

In the highlight of the above rationale, CDC encouraged the use of cloth face coverings to prevent the transmission of the virus and to protect those who might have the infection but yet not diagnosed. Cloth face masks can be easily crafted from simple household products or traditional inexpensive fabrics and can ensure superior protection in the daily lifestyle. Old scarfs, handkerchiefs, bandanas are also recommended to make masks.

Now, it is clear that the cloth face mask can provide safety from not only those who are infected but against those too who are yet to diagnose. But, CDC also emphasized the maintenance of social distancing, which in the opposite way, would cancel the effectiveness of face masks. The six feet social distancing plays a significant role in helping the virus slow down and thus should be given as much importance as face masks.

Thus, given the circumstances where people may be asymptomatic, that is to spread the virus without knowing the person has symptoms, it is highly recommended by both WHO and CDC to wear cloth face masks with the constant use of hand-sanitization and maintenance of social distancing. Only then will it limit the dissemination of the virus as well as remain safe.

China and precautionary measures

China is the main center for coronavirus, and it has successfully overcome the infection. A sharp drop can be seen in the COVID-19 cases, and the state is soon resuming the healthy lifestyle. According to the director-general of the Chinese Center for Disease Control and Prevention (CDC), one of the leading factors in battling with COVID-19 was to strictly follow precautions.

As George Gao says, the biggest mistake other countries are making is to not recommending their people to wear masks. Since there are no vaccines or antidot available, not wearing a mask simply means welcoming the disaster. There are contaminants everywhere in the air, and once these droplets reach a person's body, the virus activates. The only way to stop this dissemination is to cover the areas from where the pathogen can enter the body, that is, the mouth and the nose, and the covering can be done by face masks.

George Gao also emphasized on social distancing, saying along with the usage of masks, people should stay away at least 1 to 3 feet away from each other if the six feet apart social distancing is not possible. Face masks are necessary for everyone, as well as hand sanitization. The misunderstanding comes here where people began to replace face mask with other precautionary measures while it is clearly not effective in protection against COVID-19. The primary point to not protect others, surely it is, but first, a person should defend their own body by proper face masking, hand-washing, and social distancing.

Other countries

Following the precautions, Hong Kong, Thailand, Japan, South Korea, and several other countries have also advised their people to wear non-surgical masks, both in-home and crowded places. Thereby, assuming the protection is fulfilled by just using the face mask is wrong, but surely this tiny piece of cloth can play a significant role in this was against COVID-19.

Face mask or face covering?

There are two terms: face mask and face covering. Both are different in terms of protection, material, and preparation. A face mask is something that is worn out by a person from mouth and nose to the ears or the back of the neck. It is fixed with something, usually with elastic bands, or hooks. While on the other hand, face-covering is done by anything that is instantly used to "cover" the mouth and nose for some time. Another difference between both the terms is that face masks are usually stitched, while face coverings are held either by hands or ties. A face mask can be used for a longer time, while face covering may not be used for a longer time because it is not fixed and needs constant holding.

CHAPTER 4
FACTORS TO LOOK FOR

There are different materials that can be used to make face masks. Some are good, while some are not. Before we move on to what materials are useful and what should not be used, let's have a quick look at what are the factors that render a material better or useless.

1. Breathable

The mask should be breathable; otherwise, it will create suffocation. In other words, the mask should be dense enough to let all the impure particles out, but at the same time, it should be able to provide enough oxygen too. Breathing is vital of course, not only because it is fundamental to life, but also because if the air cannot go inside the mask, it will eventually bypass from the sides. This will create the same effect as no-masking because the air going inside the body from the sides would not be filtered, and all the pathogenic organisms would have a high chance of entering the body.

The second point of why a mask should be breathable is that other than causing the air to reach the body without filtration, it can cause suffocation, heat, or sweating. It doesn't matter how many layers are used in a mask for protection; if it cannot provide enough air to breathe, the person would be forced unconsciously to adjust the mask or remove it for some time to breathe in the open air. In both cases, the purpose of wearing a face mask would be canceled immediately.

2. Filtration power

The filtration power defines how effective a face mask is, and it depends on how dense the material is. The thicker a fabric is, the more particles will be stopped from entering the body. It also depends on the layering, sometimes there are two, and at times, even three layers are added to protect the mouth and nose. However, since this factor combines with the breathing one, the material should be dense enough to cover the face without causing much trouble.

Talking about filtration, you should not just put one layer after others and then another thinking it would be best. Instead, it is necessary to strike a balance between the two: breathing and filtration. How much convenience is it to breathe into the mask will eventually define how secure, and compelling the mask is. It will also affect the amount of time the mask will be worn. Therefore, before using any material to make a mask, try to look through it under the sun. If you feel a lot of sunlight is passing through it in, it might not be the best option. Instead, use a fabric that doesn't make a lot of light come through.

3. Face shapes

Though it is already discussed in brief, it needs more attention. Since facemasks are one approach to cover not only yourself but also the people around COVID-19 transmission, they should complete their purpose of covering the two most sensitive parts of your face: the mouth and nose. These two are highly sensitive areas as they are the open gate for pathogenic organisms. Therefore, the mask should fit against the bridge of the nose strictly and comfortably.

The upper surface of the mask should be above the nostrils, and the lower surface should be below the lower lip. Based on the shape of your face, the mask can be loose or tight. Even if the mask is just above or below the defined positions, it should and must protect many parts of the face. Regardless of the face shape, only if the lower part of the face should be covered and the above should be exposed, the mask can serve as the most exceptional protection against the on-going health crisis.

It is also recommended to first experience the material around your face by just tying it at the back of the neck to see if it covers the most part of your face, doesn't leave any open spaces, and causes any breathing problems. If it doesn't cause any hindrance, it is perfect for making a mask.

4. Ear protection

Though the main aim of a mask is to protect the mouth and nose, the ears should not be ignored in any case. Since most of the stitched masks use elastics which pass through the ears, the tension and stress in these flexible elastics can make your ears raw. Wearing a face mask for a long time can also cause irritation and redness around the ears. To avoid all these situations, it is better to use an elastic that is soft and flexible. Also, using strands is not a good option as it can cause rashes on the skin.

The other options are using those straps that can go around buttons or using hooks. You can also tie the fabric, but in that case, there are always chances of covering getting loose, so it is better to secure the mask as much as possible.

Materials: which one to go for

The following are some materials that are best for making a face mask. They fulfill the criteria that render a mask as appropriate and effective.

1. Pillowcases

Those old pillows which are mostly put in large tanks need to be taken out because pillowcases are one of the best fabrics to make masks. They have this amazing ability to filter out particles while causing no hindrance in the breathing. This is the same reason why most of us can sleep with our face pressed against the pillow surface.

Pillowcases are best because they don't cause any problems even if two layers are used in the mask, thus striking a perfect balance between breathing and filtration.

2. Flannel pajamas

Flannel is a fabric most useful to make a mask. It offers a decent filtration potential and, at the same time, doesn't allow any suffocation. Most of the times, it is used in the preparation of pajamas. So, if you have flannel pajamas in your home, you are all set because you can make really effective masks using this fabric. Plus, because the material is a bit flexible, the mask won't need an elastic, which in turn will save the ears from getting rashes.

3. Kitchen towels

Kitchen towels are another material that offers well-functioning filtration. Most of the time, they are used to clean split liquids on slabs, but they can also be used to make good masks. They are made with such a material that is soft to touch, so the mask will be great not only on keeping the pathogens out but also causing no irritation on the face. The cotton used in the kitchen towel acts as an air filter while being soft to the face.

4. Bedsheets

Bed sheets also come in the category of right materials to make homemade masks because the sheet fabric has a high thread count that can help in keeping the air particles away from mouth and nose. Any bedding item that is not stained, and is in good condition can be used well to make face masks. However, the caution requires to double-check the sheet for hygiene confirmation. In case if the bedsheet was not in use, it should be first adequately washed.

5. Quilters cotton

Now here comes the question, what exactly is quilters cotton. Quilting cotton is made from pure cotton and doesn't include any type of harmful chemicals in preparation. The fabrics made from this type of cotton are great because they are light-weight, soft to touch, and offer high-filtration against air contaminants. Any material that includes quilters cotton is an excellent option to make masks.

Materials: which one to avoid

Just like there are fabrics that are good for masks, there are also some materials that you should avoid because A, they don't offer much filtration, and B, if they do, they cause too much suffocation. So, it is better to have a look at them so that they are not used in the preparation of masks.

1. Vacuum cleaner bags

Vacuum cleaner bags are very much good for filtration purposes, but do they provide any air to breathe? The answer is no because the material used in vacuum cleaner bags is too thick that air cannot pass through them for breathing purposes. They are not recommended because they are not safe to use as they are mostly made from glass micro-fiber, which is hazardous to the respiratory system. Thus, vacuum cleaner bags should not be used in any case.

2. Old t-shirts

T-shirts are usually a decent option for mask making, but not when they are old. Since they are washed every now and then when they are in use, their material gets old and ineffective to be used. Old t-shirts may offer proper breathing but may not provide enough filtration, which nullifies the purpose of face masks. Pathogenic organisms are always ready to attach, and anything that doesn't offer proper filtration should not be used in the first place.

3. Fiberglass fabrics

You should be careful of any fabric that may contain fiberglass. As already discussed, fiberglass is dangerous to the respiratory system and causes a lot of damage if it gives high-filtration. The reason why fiberglass is not recommended is that it causes irritant contact dermatitis. In case if a person gets into too much interaction with fiberglass, they may face breathing problems or skin irritation.

4. Regular cotton

There is a difference between quilting cotton and regular cotton. The former one is good for mask masking because it is made of pure cotton. While the later one may contain some toxic synthetic chemicals which can lead to respiratory illness. Any mask made from regular cotton will contain these chemicals, and thereby, mask-making should be avoided with any fabric that is not made of organic cotton.

Emergency materials

Emergency materials are those which can be used in the instant preparation of masks. They are not actual masks; preferably, they are used as a way to cover the face in times of crisis. They offer proper filtration as well as space to breathe. They are not recommended in normal usage because they are either vulnerable or can become loose after some hours. However, in the case where no alternative to an effective mask is available, they can be used to fulfill the need of the hour.

1. Tissues

You can make a mask using a tissue paper, but as it is made from fragile material, once it gets wet, it will be of no use. Besides, they are fragile and will take no time to get teared up. However, at times of sneezing or coughing, using a tissue as a covering around the face is highly recommended. Also, the tissue should be discarded immediately without touching the used part.

2. Scarfs

Scarfs are another approach for face covering when a proper mask is not available. Most of the time, scarfs are wrapped around the mouth and nose for protection against COVID-19, but since there are no fixed elastics or hooks, they can get loose after some hours, which can create space between the mouth and the surface of the scarf. However, the material of a scarf can be used to stitch a mask too.

3. Bandanas

Unlike tissues and scarfs which are wrapped around the face, bandanas are usually tied at the backside of the neck. Bandanas are perfect to create a quick covering, but they are not advised for longer hours as they can get loose. Also, their re-adjustment will require touching the face, which, again, is not safe.

Chart on materials

Good materials	Bad materials	Emergency materials
Pillowcases	Vacuum clean bags	Tissues
T-shirts	Old t-shirts	Scarfs
Kitchen towels	Fiberglass fabrics	Bandanas
Quilters cotton	Regular cotton	
Bedsheets		
Flannel pajamas		

CHAPTER 5
STEP BY STEP TUTORIAL TO STITCH MASK

Here we are going to look deeper into how you can stitch your fabric face mask out of anything that is not harmful to the skin and lungs. You can take pillowcases, bedsheets, quilting fabric, kitchen towels, flannel pajamas, as well as any t-shirt that is not old. However, it should be noted that those fabrics which have some stretch or elasticity should be preferred for no-sew face masks. The stitching process is the same for every fabric as they require the same simple step every time.

Material required

You will need:

- Any good fabric
- Elastic

Tools required

You will need:

- Needle
- Thread

- Scissors
- Common pins
- Measuring scale
- Sewing machine (not necessary as you can also stitch it by hand)

Instructions:

1. Cut two rectangles of fabric. The measurement of each should be 10 x 6 inches. Note that this is the standard measurement for each face shape. You may add or less as per your requirement.

2. Cut two pieces of elastic. Each should be at least 6 inches. In case you don't have elastic, you can also go for hair ties, rubber bands, cloth strips, and any string.

3. Now, place one rectangular piece over the other, adjust from each side until it seems one piece. The mask is going to be stitched with two layers as one.

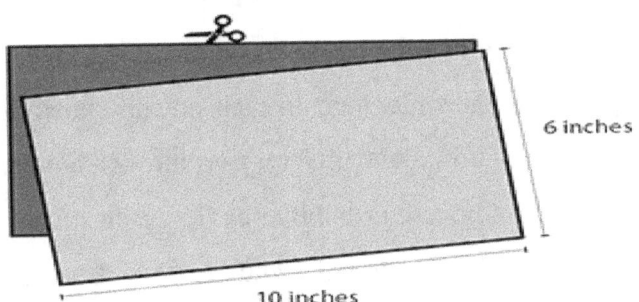

4. There are four sides of the fabric after putting both layers over each other. As illustrated in the image above, two layers are longer in length than the other two (these are 10 inches sides). Fold over the longer sides for about ¼ inch. Use common pins to secure them.

5. Then hem both sides either by using a sewing machine, or you can also do it with your own hands.

6. Now you have two sides of the fabric stitched, while two short sides are still unstitched (these are 6 inches sides). Just like the longer layers, fold over the short sides for about ½ inch and secure them with common pins. Then stitch them.

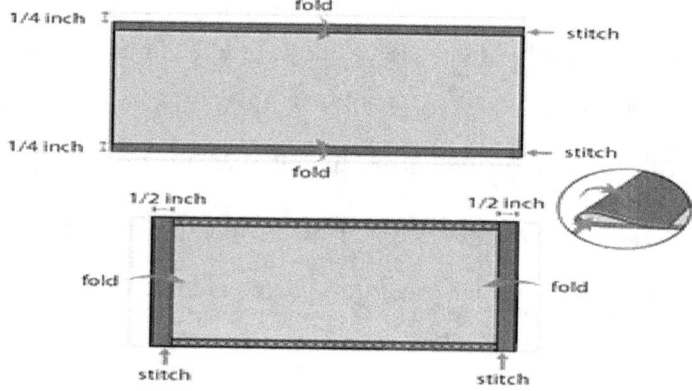

7. After stitching all sides successfully, it is time to use elastic pieces. In the wider hem on each side (as shown in the circle on the right of above image), pass through a piece of elastic by using a pencil, or bobby pin. The easiest way to do is to attach a safety pin with one end of elastic. Running the safety pin through the wider hem will systematically take elastic

with it.

8. Do the same with the other side. The process will be the same in case you are using cloth strips, rubber bands, or hair ties.

9. Tightly knot the two ends of one elastic on one side of the fabric, or as shown in the image below. Repeat the same with the other elastic string.

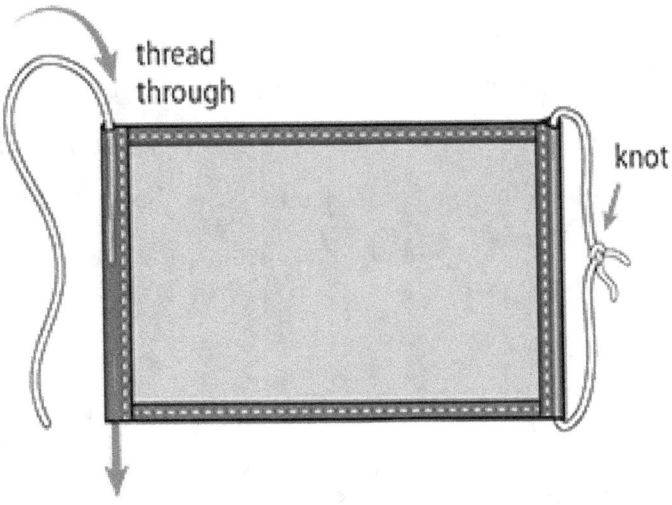

10. This step requires adjustment of the mask according to your face shape. After knotting each elastic band, pull them. Make sure to do this gently; otherwise the elastic may break or become too much loose. Tuck the knots inside the hem so that they don't tease when you wear the mask.

11. Now, try to put the mask over your face and the elastics over the ears to see if the mask fits perfectly or not. Remember, the purpose of the mask is to cover your mouth and nose, and thus the upper surface of the mask should be above the

nostrils, and the lower surface should be below the lower lip. Also, the mask should fit against the bridge of the nose tightly.

12. At this step, stitch the elastic on each side of the hem. It will keep it in place so that it does not slip. Also, before stitching, ensure that the notes are inside the hem area. In case the mask doesn't fit your face or is loose, you can run more elastic through the wider hem and then stitch to shorten the elastic that will go over your ears. While if the elastic is too tight, you may open the knot and loose it a bit, or if possible, use another piece of elastic. After the mask fully fits your face, stitch it with the knot inside the hem area, or as shown here.

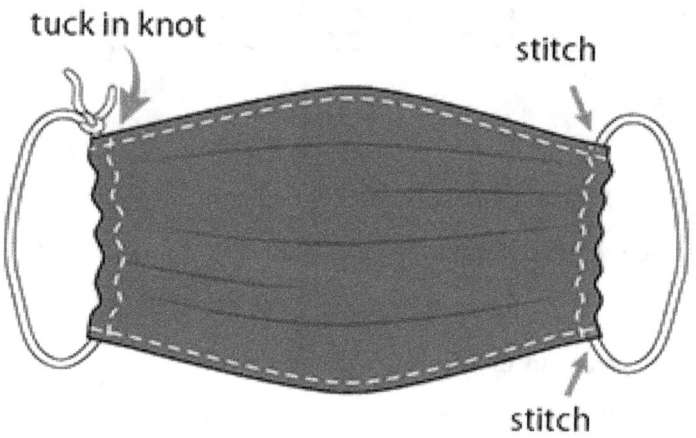

Your mask is ready!

Step by Step tutorials to make a no-sew mask

If you don't want to stitch a mask, you can also make with fewer efforts. While fabrics such as bedsheets, pillowcases, and kitchen towels come in stitching category, t-shirts, flannel pajamas, and bandanas can be used to make quick masks. It is noteworthy that these masks are not created by wrapping around the face in emergency cases. Instead, they are correctly measured and thus require the same attention and care as stitched masks.

1. T-shirt / Flannel pajama mask

T-shirts are perfect for making a non-stitched mask. These masks are quick, flexible, and easy to use. One thing to make sure that the t-shirt to be used should not be too old, as it won't be beneficial. If the t-shirt is cleaned from any stains and is in good condition, then it is good to go. The procedure is the same with flannel pajama. Here we have used the illustrations with a t-shirt because not everyone has flannel pajamas in their home. However, the steps are the same and can be adjusted accordingly.

Materials required

You will need

- A t-shirt that is not very old

Tools required

- Scissors
- Chalk or pen
- Measuring scale

Instructions

1. Even if the t-shirt is in good condition, it is always recommended to wash it before use. The reason is that t-shirts, unlike bedsheets or pillow fabrics, are most exposed to the air contaminants. Therefore, it is better to clean them before they are used as a mask.

2. After the t-shirt is washed and dried, lay it on a flat surface and remove any creases. This is important because the t-shirt is made of stretchy material, and not eliminating any creases can lead to wrong measurements and uneven mask.

3. Cut a 7 to 8 inches apart from the bottom side of the t-shirt, while making sure the length on both sides is equal. Remember, this measurement is for a standard-sized t-shirt, and the mask you are going to make will depend on the

horizontal length of your t-shirt. Do, as illustrated below.

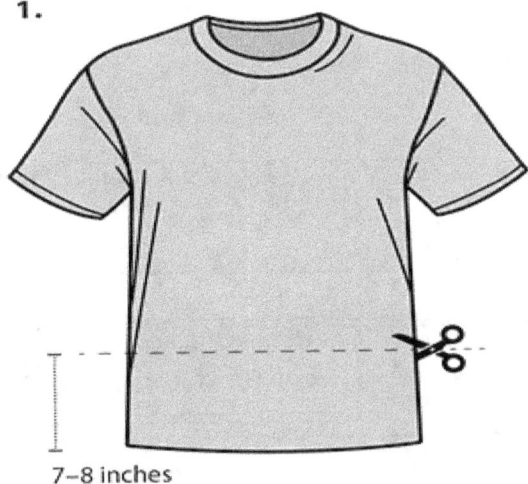

4. Now, take the piece you have cut and again lay it on the flat surface. Remove any creases. By using chalk or pen, draw a 6 inches rectangle in the horizontal shape on the right side of the piece. Make sure to leave at least 1 or 2 inches from both up and below surfaces. Now take the scissor and cut the rectangle.

5. Next, leave the cut part aside, and by using a scissor, cut the upper and lower corners of the piece so that they can be tied later.

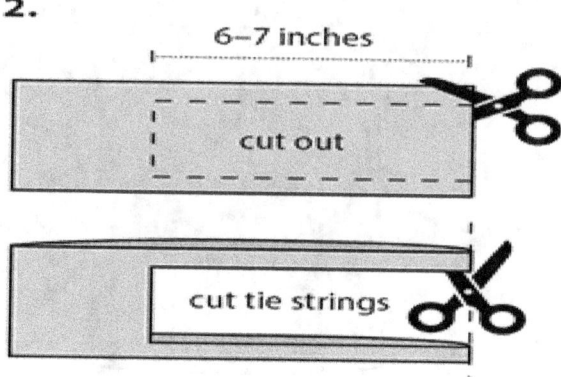

6. Here you have to adjust the face mask. Since the t-shirt is not old, a single layer would offer enough protection. Try to lift the mask and cover your face with it to see if the mask adjusts right. Since such masks are tied, and no elastics are used, they cause less irritation and problems.

7. See how long the strings are required. If they are short, you can cut one more inch in 4rth step. If they are too long, you can cut the excess.

8. Once the strings are in the perfect length, cover your face with the mask and first tie the lower end around the neck, then tie the upper string over the top of the head. And you are good to go with your mask!

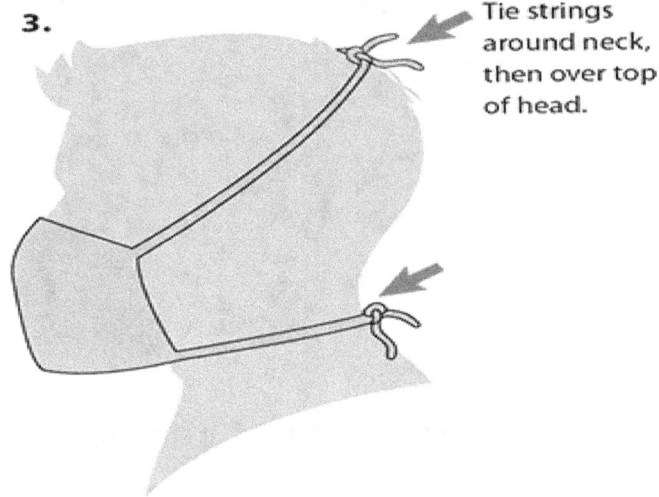

2 Bandana face mask

Bandana face masks are also one of the effective and quick, no-sew masks that can be used as protection against COVID-19. Like a scarf, bandana fabric can be wrapped around the face to cover it. However, in case you want to make a proper face mask, the procedure is easy and quick. In fact, having the right measurements, it would not be wrong to say that a bandana mask can be made in less than one minute.

Materials required

- A bandana
- Rubber bands

Tools required

- Scissors
- Chalk or pen
- Measuring scale

Instructions

1. Take the bandana and lay it on a flat surface to remove any creases. Cut out a square of 20 x 20 inches.

2. By using the measuring scale and pen, mark on the middle of the cloth, which is 10 inches. Fold the fabric in half from upside down.

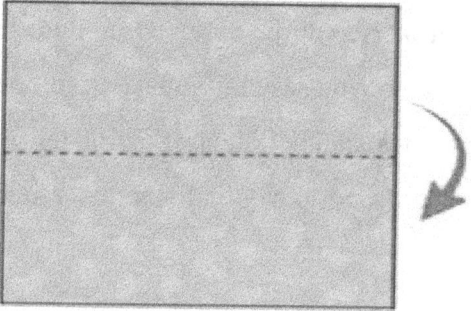

3. Next, again by using the measuring scale and pen, mark three equal parts of the cloth and fold the upper and lower layer in such a way that one layer comes above the other. The measurements should be carefully made to avoid any mistakes. All you have to do is to first fold the top down and

then the bottom up, or as shown here.

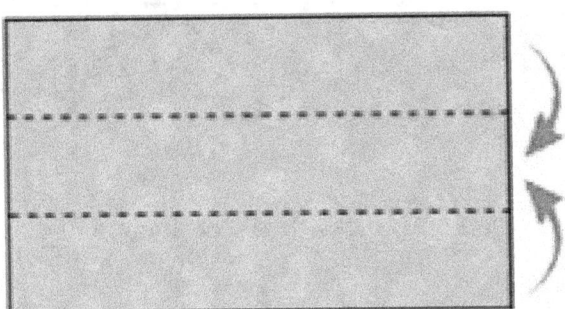

4   Now, it is time to use rubber bands. If you don't have rubber bands, you can also use hair ties. You can also use elastic bands, but for that, you first have to tie a knot. Take the rubber bands and pass them through each side. The distance between both should be at least 6 inches.

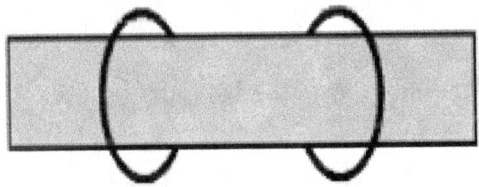

5   It is better to mark the right positions of rubber bands. Fold both sides of bandana cloth exact at where the rubber ties are. Once they are folded, tuck one side in the other.

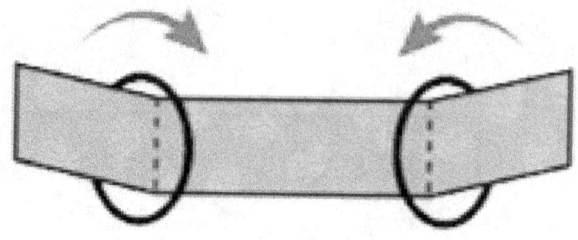

6   After you have tucked the sides, you will get the following shape:

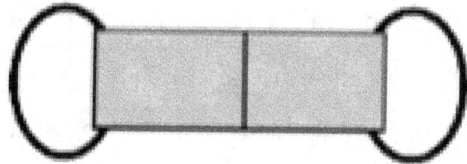

7   In the last step, take the mask to your face, slip one loop over one ear, and the other loop over the other ear. Adjust it to fit your face. And your quick bandana face mask is ready!

Bandana face mask using a coffee filter

To increase the effectiveness of a bandana face mask, you can add a coffee filter inside the layers. Unlike the vacuum cleaner bag, the coffee filter is useful in preventing the microorganisms from reaching the mouth and nose. It has no fiberglass, which makes it better than vacuum filtration.

The steps are the same as a bandana face mask. Just before the folding step, which is the very first step, you have to cut out the coffee filter, and later in the second folding, place the coffee filter in the fabric.

- Take the coffee filter and cut it in half.

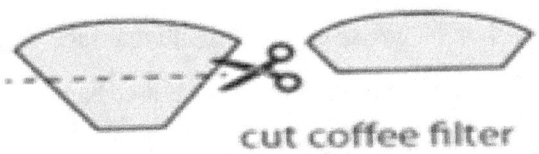

cut coffee filter

- Next, fold the fabric in half. Just before folding it into the top down and bottom left, put the coffee filter in the middle section like this:

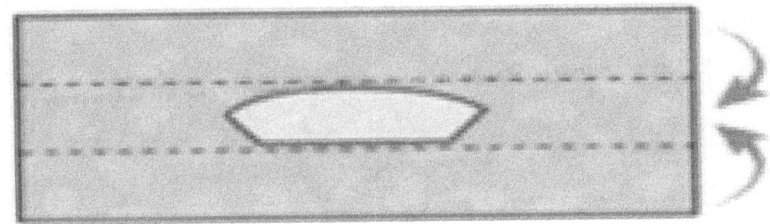

- Now, repeat all the steps as making a bandana face mask!

Important notes

- By using the same step-by-step method as a bandana face mask, any fabric can be used to make a mask. The only thing to make sure is the right measurement that, in case of any fabric, will be 20 x 20 inches. People are encouraged to wear scarfs in the same way a bandana mask is worn to ensure maximum protection. Also, the coffee filter can be used in a fabric face mask, too, by putting it in the center of the folded fabric piece.

- Rubber bands are used in a bandana face mask, but if possible, try to use hair ties. As rubber bands are made of strong elastic, they are often harsh against the soft skin of ears as well as the cheeks. Hair ties, on the other hand, are less rough than rubber bands and often contain the soft layers, which will help keep the ears from irritation.

CHAPTER 6
WHAT IS THE PROPER WAY TO WEAR A MASK?

Follow these steps:

- The first step is to clean your hands with soap and water for at least a minute with the right actions.

- Next, put on a hand-sanitizer and rub your hands against each other.

- Clearly examine the mask for any fault. It can include teared up material or broken elastics. If the mask is in a fine position, it is good to be used.

- Hold the mask to your face in a straight position.

- You can slip the loops directly in your ears, but to make the mask tighter and less-spacy, you can twist the rubber band, elastic, or hair tie and then wear it. The same goes for the other loop.

- Adjust the mask. Adjustment is always necessary to make sure the mask is not too tight or too loose as the right fit will lessen the chances of touching the face. Remember, if you touch your face, you cancel the purpose of the mask; therefore, adjust it properly. If you have twisted the loops, and the mask feels too close, untwist them. While if the mask feels too loose, you can twist the ear loops again to make it fit for your face.

- Also, make sure that the mask is in the right position, that it is well covering your mouth and nose as well as the upper surface is mounted against your nose bridge.

- Once the mask is worn out, do not touch the front part in any case. If it gets wet, or defected, dispose of it immediately.

What is the proper way to un-wear a mask?

- Make sure to wash the hands properly with soap and water for at least one minute with proper washing actions.

- After that, sanitize the hands with an alcohol-based hand sanitizer.

- Since the mask has been used, its front part would be full of pollutants and contaminants, so avoid touching it. Instead, hold the mask from the elastics at the back of the ears.

- Gently pull the loops over the ears and carefully remove the mask without letting your hands touch its surface.

- Carefully hold the loops in your hands and dispose of the mask instantly in the bin. In case it is washable, wash it carefully.

- Again, wash your hands with soap and water, and sanitize

them properly before putting another mask.

Common mistakes about masks

1 Thinking not wearing a mask is okay!

No, it is not Okay at all! Not wearing a mask means allowing pathogenic organisms to enter your body. It also means opening the door of infection and then infecting others. So, wearing a mask is a must.

2 Occasionally wearing a mask

If there is the danger of COVID-19, the mask should be worn over all the time. You should not do what some people do, and that is to wear a mask one day and then to live other days as if there is no danger out there.

3 Not washing hands before or after using a mask

Hand washing is necessary, and so the hand sanitization. Whenever you wear a mask, use proper actions to clean your hands to make sure there is no impurity left. The same goes for the other side, that you should and must wash your hands after you dispose of a used mask. As there are always contaminants in the air, it is important to ensure hygiene for the protection against COVID-19.

4 Wearing loose masks

The mask should cover almost half of your face, and for that, it is vital that the surface of the mask should touch your skin. Otherwise, the dangerous particles can reach your mouth from the spaces between the mask surface and skin. To avoid this, make sure the mask fits properly around the nose and mouth.

5 Wearing too tight masks

Though it is contrary to the above point, it requires the same attention. The mask you would wear should not be too tight around your face as one objective of the mask is to allow air for breathing while protecting. If the mask is extra fitted, the less-air for breathing can cause suffocation. It is hard to wear a mask when a person is feeling suffocation, and touching the mask to adjust will, in turn, nullify the actual purpose. The rule of thumb is to use a mask that is not too tight nor too loose and fits appropriately.

6 Touching the mask after wearing it

Now, this is another common mistake people make. Keep in mind that once the mask is worn over, it should not be touched in any case. The one purpose of the mask is to limit the touching of the mouth and nose. While the hands are touched everywhere, they are most exposed to pathogens and viruses. What is recommended is to properly wear a mask at once so that later adjustments can be prevented.

7 Un-wearing the face mask from the front part

No, it is, again, strictly prohibited. It is more dangerous, especially if the mask is worn over for a day. Still, regardless of time, you should remove a mask by using loops only and also dispose of a mask by holding the loops only. Since the loops are less exposed, they have fewer particles as compared to the front part.

8 Hanging the mask around the neck

A person should never do it, not even for fun. A mask is meant to protect the mouth and nose, and not to be hanged on the neck. In order to ensure the safety, a mask should be worn over the half of the face.

9 Hanging the mask from one ear

Don't let a mask hang in one ear as it can be contaminated. Just like hanging the mask in the neck, it is risky and unsafe to dangle the mask from the ear and should be prevented.

10 Reusing a mask without washing it properly

After a single-use, the mask becomes contaminated. It should be cleaned before reusing it. Not washing a used mask simply means putting all the microorganisms again on your face and letting them enter the body. Thereby, always properly clean a reusable mask. Also, wash your hands before and after cleaning a mask.

Frequently Asked Questions regarding masks

1 Should a face mask cover the chin?

There is no limitation, but covering the chin is not necessarily important too. As the main areas to cover are the mouth and nose, not covering the chin will not affect in a negative way. However, it can be useful as a good seal around the mouth and nose can be obtained by wearing a mask that also covers chin.

2 How to touch mask after wearing it?

Though touching the mask is not recommended in any situation, if there is no other alternative, wash your hands and sanitize them properly before and after touching it.

3 How frequently should the mask be replaced?

If it is a disposable mask, it should be discarded immediately. While in the case of reusable masks, they should be washed after each time they are used. If they are used in the home, then every day, and if they are worn over in a public place, then the masks should be washed right after the visit.

4 What to do if the ears get rashes or redness?

While wearing masks, it is common to get skin-irritation because the surface of the mask and the elastics are constantly being dragged against the skin—the best way to avoid it to use a mask with buttons at the back of the head. Hooks are also a good option, and they come with an S-ring to be hooked at the back of the neck.

5 What are the places you should wear a mask?

Whenever you go out to any public place, you should wear a mask. Whether it is a grocery store, pharmacy, or even while walking on a street, you should not forget the mask. The use of the mask is a must in those places which are crowded and where six feet apart social distancing is nearly impossible.

6 What about the small gaps in masks?

A face mask is like a shield over the face, and any holes in that shield can be risky. Spaces are dangerous because they allow the passage of contaminants. However, since it is not possible to eliminate the spaces completely, what should be kept in mind to limit the gaps between the face and the mask. The fewer the gaps are, the lesser is the danger.

7 Which one is better: stitched or non-stitched masks?

The stitched ones are better. The non-stitched can lose their shape because they are not fixed by anything like a thread. However, if talk about the effectivity, both types provide equal protection against coronavirus. Just that non-stitched masks are quick and easy to make but are less durable while stitched face masks take some time and don't get in bad condition for long.

8 Should you wear a mask at home?

The answer is tricky, as it depends on how many people live in a house or room. There is no need to wear a mask at home if every person inside the house is in a healthy condition. However, in case anyone has caught flu, or fever, you should wear a mask at home with proper hand-sanitization.

9 What if you have to un-wear a mask?

You cannot wear a mask for hours, and even if it does happen, there are always situations when you have to take off the mask, such as eating. It is recommended to use a designated brown paper bag to store the face mask. Of-course if it is a disposable mask, it should be thrown in the bin, while in case of cloth face mask, it can be placed in a brown paper bag. Also, it is recommended to change the paper bag daily.

10 What are the quick dos and don'ts of wearing masks?

Wear a mask while going out. Wash and sanitize hands before and after using a mask. Do not touch the front part of the mask. Do not wear a loose or tight face mask. Use a mask that allows comfort at breathing and protection at the same time. Wash the cloth face mask everyday in-home and every time after a visit to the outer world.

Bottom line

Coronavirus was originated in Wuhan, but the whole world is affected by it. Hundreds and thousands of innocent people have died, and half of the humanity is destroyed just because of a tiny, but extremely dangerous microorganism. The number of cases is increasing; the deaths have reached an alarming rate, and this health crisis has destroyed almost everything on our planet. The need of the hour is not to lament, but to think of the ways that can save the mother earth, and thereby, humanity.

Everyone is in a constant state of panic. What should be in focus right now is how we can put a stop on it. It is not impossible, and who knows the cost of getting back to a healthy world may take more hundreds and thousands of lives. But that doesn't mean it should be left alone. Though we don't have any vaccine or antidote against it, we do have precautionary measures to help us combat this curse.

It is vital to sort out the priorities, and on the top of the list should be to stay safe and keep others safe. Thereby, using facemasks is an urgent necessity to not only protect us but everyone out there. And along with that, proper hand sanitization, and social distancing matter the same. Following all these three vital objectives can reduce the chances of getting infected. The world is in danger, and every human should play its role in saving it. By virtue of the fact, keep following precautions, for they are our only weapons!

REFERENCES

1. MacIntyre, C. R., & Chughtai, A. A. (2015). Facemasks for the prevention of infection in healthcare and community settings. Bmj, 350, h694.

2. Davies, A., Thompson, K. A., Giri, K., Kafatos, G., Walker, J., & Bennett, A. (2013). Testing the efficacy of homemade masks: would they protect in an influenza pandemic? Disaster medicine and public health preparedness, 7(4), 413-418.

3. Coronavirus Disease 2019 (COVID-19) – Prevention & Treatment. (2020). Retrieved 7 May 2020, from https://www.cdc.gov/coronavirus/2019-ncov/prevent-getting-sick/prevention.html

4. Coronavirus Disease 2019 (COVID-19). (2020). Retrieved 7 May 2020, from https://www.cdc.gov/coronavirus/2019-ncov/prevent-getting-sick/cloth-face-cover.html

5. When and how to use masks. (2020). Retrieved 7 May 2020, from https://www.who.int/emergencies/diseases/novel-coronavirus-2019/advice-for-public/when-and-how-to-use-masks

6. Coronavirus Disease 2019 (COVID-19). (2020). Retrieved 7 May 2020, from https://www.cdc.gov/coronavirus/2019-ncov/prevent-getting-sick/cloth-face-cover.html

7. Not wearing masks to protect against coronavirus is a 'big mistake,' top Chinese scientist says. (2020). Retrieved 7 May 2020, from https://www.sciencemag.org/news/2020/03/not-wearing-masks-protect-against-coronavirus-big-mistake-top-chinese-scientist-says#

www.ingramcontent.com/pod-product-compliance
Lightning Source LLC
Chambersburg PA
CBHW070317220526
45465CB00004B/1879